# Adrenal Insufficiency 101

# A Patient's Guide to Managing Adrenal Insufficiency
### Second Edition

By: Winslow E. Dixon
Founder/Former CEO of
Adrenal Alternatives Foundation

This book was written from a patient's perspective and is not intended to give or replace medical care, advice or provide treatment of any medical condition.

ISBN: 978-1-7349073-0-8

Printed in the United States of America.

Second printing edition: December 2023.

# Table of Contents

# Chapter 1:
# Understanding the Adrenals

## Introduction

Adrenal insufficiency is a condition where the adrenal glands fail to produce the proper amounts of steroid hormone(s). There are many different forms of adrenal disease, but the treatment for all forms is the same, steroids for hormone replacement.

In a normal person, during situations of emotional or physical stress their body releases more cortisol. The excitement from a happy event, the sadness from a death of a loved one or the strain from exercising are examples of things that would cause the body to release more cortisol. In an adrenal insufficient person, this does not happen. When someone has adrenal insufficiency, they are faced with the task of not only replacing a life-sustaining hormone, but also replicating a failed body system. Artificially managing cortisol is a complex task and is vital to quality of life. An adrenal patient's personal cortisol needs may differ from day to day depending on physical, emotional and environmental stressors.

## Terms to Know

Adrenocorticotropic hormone (ACTH) - Polypeptide tropic hormone which is crucial in the hypothalamic-pituitary-adrenal axis. ACTH is produced by the anterior pituitary gland and stimulates the adrenal glands to produce cortisol.

Aldosterone (ALD)- Mineralocorticoid hormone which regulates electrolyte balances by instructing the kidneys to release potassium and retain sodium. It also helps regulate blood pressure.

Adrenal Insufficiency- Condition which results in the lack of cortisol production and can also result in lack of DHEA, aldosterone and disrupt the balance of the immune system, inflammation levels, endocrine hormones, electrolyte homeostasis, sodium and potassium levels and also can impact blood pressure and body temperature regulation. There are many forms of adrenal insufficiency.

Adrenal glands- Walnut shaped glands located on top of each kidney which produce cortisol. catecholamines, DHEA and androgenic steroids. The adrenal gland is comprised of two parts:
1-Adrenal medulla- The inner part of an adrenal gland which controls hormones epinephrine (adrenaline) and norepinephrine (noradrenaline).
2- Adrenal cortex- The outer part of the gland that produces hormones such as cortisol and aldosterone.

Catecholamines- Hormones such as dopamine, epinephrine (adrenaline) and norepinephrine (noradrenaline) that the adrenals produce in response to physical or emotional stress by increasing heart rate and blood pressure.

Cortisol– Glucocorticoid hormone: The body's stress hormone that is produced by the zona fasciculata. It helps control the body's use of fats, proteins and carbohydrates; suppresses inflammation, impacts blood pressure and blood sugar. It also controls the body's sleep/wake cycle and impacts the circadian rhythm.

Circadian rhythm- The body's natural, internal process that regulates the sleep-wake cycle and repeats roughly every 24 hours. Circadian rhythms can be physical, mental, and behavioral patterns that follow a daily cycle. Cortisol is deeply crucial to circadian rhythm modulation.

CRH (corticotropin-releasing hormone)- A peptide hormone which the signals the pituitary synthesis of ACTH (Adrenocorticotropic hormone).

DHEA– Hormone that aids in the production of androgens and estrogens (male and female sex hormones)

Glucocorticoids- Corticosteroid hormones that bind to glucocorticoid receptors and are part of the feedback mechanism in the immune system which reduces certain aspects of immune function, such as inflammation.

Mineralocorticoids- Corticosteroids that regulate electrolyte balance and fluid balance in the body.  In salt wasting forms of adrenal disease, mineralocorticoid replacement is necessary. Medications such as fludrocortisone are used to supplement mineralocorticoid deficiency.

17-Hydroxyprogesterone- Endogenous progestogen steroid hormone related to progesterone which is critical in the biosynthesis of androgens, estrogens, glucocorticoids, and mineralocorticoids.

### Diseases/Conditions impacting the Adrenal Glands[1]

Adrenal adenoma- Benign tumor of the adrenal glands, which can lead to overproduction of the adrenal hormones.

---

[1] TYPES OF ADRENAL GLAND DISORDERS
https://www.nichd.nih.gov/. (2020). Types of adrenal gland disorders. [online] Available at:
https://www.nichd.nih.gov/health/topics/adrenalgland/conditioninfo/types

Addison's disease- Autoimmune disease resulting in the destruction of the adrenal glands, rendering them unable to produce proper amounts of cortisol, DHEA & Aldosterone.

Adrenocortical Carcinoma- Cancerous adrenal tumor that tends to develop in the outer layer of the adrenal gland.

Conn's syndrome- Rare health condition which results in the adrenal glands producing too much aldosterone, also known as primary hyperaldosteronism.

Congenital adrenal hyperplasia (CAH)- Genetic disorder present from birth that impairs the adrenal glands. CAH patients lack the enzymes the adrenal glands use to produce hormones that help regulate metabolism, the immune system, blood pressure and other essential functions.

There are two main types of congenital adrenal hyperplasia—classic and nonclassic. The majority of people diagnosed with this condition do not produce enough 21-hydroxylase, which is the enzyme that helps the adrenal glands make cortisol and aldosterone.

There are also other much rarer forms of CAH such as:

11-Beta hydroxylase deficiency- Form of CAH which can be present in both genders, but in females with the non-classic form of CAH, they may develop excessive body hair growth (hirsutism) and irregular menstruation. Males with this condition do not typically have any signs or symptoms except for small height.

17a-hydroxylase deficiency- Form of CAH which results from a defect in the gene CYP17A1, which encodes for the enzyme 17a-hydroxylase. This causes decreased synthesis of cortisol and sex steroids. Can present with ambiguous genitalia in genetic males and also cause failure of the ovaries to function at puberty in genetic females, resulting in infertility.

3-Beta-hydroxysteroid dehydrogenase deficiency- There are three types of 3BHSD deficiency, the salt-wasting form, non-salt-wasting form, and non-classic form. Males with this condition often present with abnormal external genitalia and suffer from infertility. Females with this deficiency may present with slight genital abnormalities at birth, irregular menstruation, hirsutism, and infertility. 3BHSD deficiency is caused by mutations in the HSD3B2 gene.

Congenital lipoid adrenal hyperplasia- This condition is the most severe form of CAH and may cause early death due to adrenal crisis. In this disorder, the synthesis of all adrenal and gonadal steroid hormones is impaired due to a molecular defect in the steroidogenic acute regulatory protein.  Presents in males with ambiguous genitalia.

PORD (P450 oxidoreductase deficiency) – A disorder of steroidogenesis with a broad phenotypic spectrum including cortisol deficiency, altered sex steroid synthesis and disorders of sexual development. Associated cases have been also been linked with a skeletal disorder known as Antley-Bixler syndrome.

Cushing's disease -When the pituitary gland releases too much adrenocorticotropic hormone (ACTH) resulting in the over production of the hormone, cortisol.

Hypopituitarism- Disorder in which the pituitary gland fails to produce the appropriate amount of hormones, requiring hormone replacement therapy.

May impact one or more of the following hormones:
- Adrenocorticotropic hormone (ACTH) Signals the adrenal gland to release cortisol.
- Antidiuretic hormone (ADH) Regulates water loss by the kidneys.
- Follicle-stimulating hormone (FSH) Regulates sexual function and fertility in males and females.
- Growth hormone (GH) Regulates growth of tissues and bone.
- Luteinizing hormone (LH) Regulates sexual function and fertility in males and females.
- Oxytocin- Signals the uterus to contract during labor and the breasts to release milk.
- Prolactin- Signals female breast development and milk production.
- Thyroid-stimulating hormone (TSH) Signals the thyroid gland to release hormones that affect the body's metabolism.

Pheochromocytoma- A rare tumor of adrenal gland tissue which results in the release of too much epinephrine and norepinephrine.

Secondary Adrenal Insufficiency- When the pituitary gland does not produce the hormone ATCH (Adrenocorticotropic hormone) resulting in the lack of cortisol production in the adrenal glands. Can be caused by a variety of facts such as, but not limited to hypopituitarism, exogenous steroid suppression and pituitary gland tumors.

Sheehan's syndrome- A condition that affects women during or after childbirth, which causes damage to the pituitary gland causing it to fail to produce enough pituitary hormones, also referred to as postpartum hypopituitarism.

Tertiary Adrenal Insufficiency- When the hypothalamus fails to release CRH (corticotropin-releasing hormone) which stimulates the production of ACTH by the pituitary gland.

Lymphocytic Lypophysitis- Condition in which the pituitary gland becomes damaged by lymphocytes, resulting in pituitary enlargement and impaired function.

### Possible Symptoms of Adrenal Disease

It is important to note that adrenal disease, having many forms and causes, may present differently in each case, making it difficult to suspect based on symptoms alone. However, salt cravings and fatigue seem to be present in the majority of cases.

Other possible symptoms of undiagnosed adrenal insufficiency are[2]:

(This is not an all-inclusive list and not to be used to diagnose or replace medical care)
- Anxiety
- Changes in mental status
- Fatigue
- Gastrointestinal symptoms such as nausea and vomiting
- Headaches
- Hyperpigmentation (Also known as the "addy tan")
- Low Blood Pressure
- Muscle Pain

---

[2] H., Diseases, E., Disease, A., Causes, S., Causes, S., Center, T. and Health, N. (2020). U.S. Department of Health and Human Services. [online] National Institute of Diabetes and Digestive and Kidney Diseases. Available at: https://www.niddk.nih.gov/health-information/endocrine-diseases/adrenal-insufficiency-addisons-disease/symptoms-causes.

- Muscle Weakness
- Salt Cravings
- Weakness
- Weight loss

Unfortunately, some cases of adrenal insufficiency are not diagnosed until after an adrenal crisis has occurred. An adrenal crisis is a serious event and will lead to death if left untreated. The body cannot sustain life without cortisol. If you suspect you are having adrenal issues, please get the proper testing. Early detection can prevent damage to your body and make your prognosis with adrenal insufficiency better.

### Diagnostic Testing for Adrenal Disease[3]

8 am Cortisol Blood Lab- Your body's natural cortisol levels should be the highest in the morning, according to your body's circadian rhythm. If your AM levels are low, it can indicate an adrenal issue. This test will measure the level of cortisol in your blood.

ACTH Stimulation Test- Measures how well the adrenal glands respond to the release of the adrenocorticotropic hormone (ACTH). When this test is done, your blood is drawn prior to injection of ACTH then at timed intervals to test your adrenal's response to the ACTH. If your cortisol levels do not rise properly, you are then diagnosed with adrenal insufficiency.

---

[3] TOFT MD, D. J.
Addison's Disease Diagnosis: (Toft MD, n.d.): Toft MD, D. (n.d.). Addison's Disease Diagnosis. [online] EndocrineWeb. Available at: https://www.endocrineweb.com/conditions/addisons-disease/addison-disease-diagnosis.

Aldosterone Blood Lab- Blood test which measures the amount of aldosterone (ALD) in your blood. Physicians usually test your levels of renin and aldosterone simultaneously. (Also known as a plasma renin activity test or an aldosterone-renin ratio.)

CRH Stimulation Test- Test which can help evaluate adrenal hormones by differentiating hypercortisolemia associated with Cushing's syndrome. CRH (corticotropin-releasing hormone) is a naturally occurring hormone which causes the pituitary gland to secrete the hormone ACTH.

Dexamethasone Suppression Test- Test which is primarily used to diagnose Cushing's syndrome by measuring the response of the adrenal glands to ACTH. Cortisol levels should decrease in response to the administration of dexamethasone. This test works to assess the pituitary's response to glucocorticoid negative feedback inhibition of ACTH secretion.

DHEA Blood Lab- Test which measures the blood level of dehydroepiandrosterone (DHEA) and dehydroepiandrosterone sulfate (DHEA-S).

Insulin Tolerance Test (ITT)- A test where insulin is injected into a patient's vein, after which blood glucose is measured at regular intervals used to assess adrenal function, insulin sensitivity, and pituitary function. This test is considered the standard for diagnosing growth hormone (GH) deficiency and cortisol production in pituitary assessment.

Metyrapone Test- Diagnostic test which is based upon the idea that decreasing serum cortisol concentrations normally produces an increase in ACTH secretion due to a decrease in glucocorticoid negative feedback. The test is performed primarily to detect partial defects in pituitary ACTH secretion. This test is performed when Metyrapone is introduced into the body causing the block of the conversion of 11-deoxycortisol to cortisol by CYP11B1 (11-beta-hydroxylase, P450c11) the final step in the synthesis of cortisol. This causes a decrease of cortisol and increases 11-deoxycortisol. This test is used to evaluate the hypothalamic-pituitary-adrenal axis.

Renin Blood Lab- Test which measures the level of renin in blood. A high level of renin may be indicative that the adrenal glands are not making sufficient hormones. Physicians usually test your levels of renin and aldosterone simultaneously.  (Also known as a plasma renin activity test or an aldosterone-renin ratio)

Saliva Cortisol Test- Test which measures plasma free cortisol concentration in human saliva.

Urine Cortisol Test- Also called a urinary free cortisol (UFC) test. This test measures the total amount of cortisol excreted into urine over 24 hours.

It is important to appropriately evaluate the results of blood, saliva and urine testing. There is a difference between bound cortisol and free cortisol within the body. Testing metabolized cortisol evaluates how much cortisol is being created and cleared through the liver. Testing free cortisol evaluates how much cortisol is free to bind to receptors and allows for assessment of the circadian rhythm.  The largest amount of cortisol in the body is bound to cortisol-binding globulin (CBG) and albumin. On average, less than 5% of circulating cortisol is unbound (free). Only unbound (free) cortisol can access the transporters in tissues that regulate metabolic and excretory clearance.

A small part of cortisol in the body is free. This amount of cortisol is vital, but levels of metabolized cortisol are the best evaluation of overall production of cortisol. Measuring both free and bound cortisol may provide a vital insight into the amount of cortisol metabolism and production.

It is also important to note that if adrenal insufficiency is suspected and a patient is presenting with symptoms of an adrenal crisis, standard treatment protocol of administration of steroid cortisol replacement should not be withheld due to pending lab results. If left untreated, an adrenal crisis will result in death. The body cannot survive without sufficient amounts of cortisol.

Adrenal insufficiency requires life-long cortisol replacement therapy in the form of steroid medication management. Some forms of adrenal insufficiency also require replacement of aldosterone and DHEA.

Finding the right steroid is dependent on each adrenal insufficient patient. Variables like personal cortisol clearance rates, pain levels, health comorbidities, weight, stress management and physical activity will impact dosing needs. It is important to work with an endocrinologist who is proficient in managing adrenal disease to determine the most optimal steroid replacement medication.

## Standard Treatments for Adrenal Insufficiency

The following list are the oral medications commonly prescribed for Adrenal Insufficiency[4]

---

[4] PREDNISONE AND OTHER CORTICOSTEROIDS: BALANCE THE RISKS AND BENEFITS Mayo Clinic. (2020). Prednisone and other corticosteroids: Balance the risks and benefits. [online] Available at: https://www.mayoclinic.org/steroids/art-20045692.

This is not an all-inclusive list and not to be used to diagnose or replace medical care.

Cortisone Acetate- The acetate salt form of cortisone, a synthetic or semisynthetic analog of the naturally occurring cortisone hormone. Cortisone itself is inactive; it is converted in the liver to the active metabolite hydrocortisone.

Dexamethasone (Decadron)- Medication is used in the treatment of cancers such as leukemias, and lymphomas and to treat diseases involving destruction by the body's own immune system. Also used to treat adrenal insufficiency. Dexamethasone is a long acting steroid and remains in blood circulation for approximately 16 hours after administration, with a half-life of about 4 hours.

Fludrocortisone (Florinef) – Synthetic medication used to treat salt wasting diseases such as primary Addison's disease. Fludrocortisone cannot be converted to another corticosteroid on the basis of anti-inflammatory potency. It is not a replacement for cortisol but is used in addition to cortisol replacement in some forms of adrenal disease.

Hydrocortisone (Cortef) - Medication is the most bio-identical form of cortisol. It is a short acting steroid used to treat autoimmune diseases, allergic reactions and also adrenal insufficiency. The pharmaceutical properties of the dosage of hydrocortisone are determined by intestinal absorption rate and the plasma concentration-time profile of hydrocortisone (cortisol) in a specific patient's body. There are many factors that cause or result in pharmacokinetic variability; therefore, the short elimination half-life of hydrocortisone is approximately 1.5 hours when given in traditional immediate-release dosage forms.

Methylprednisolone (Medrol)- Medication which is a synthetic corticosteroid and is mainly used to achieve prompt suppression of inflammation but can also be used to treat adrenal insufficiency.

Prednisolone (Prelone)- Synthetic glucocorticoid replacement medication used to treat adrenal insufficiency and also used to treat autoimmune diseases and allergic reactions.

Prednisone- Synthetic corticosteroid which mimics the action of cortisol produced in the body by the adrenal glands. Most often used for its potent anti-inflammatory effects, particularly in autoimmune and inflammatory diseases and conditions. Also used to treat adrenal insufficiency.

Prednisone is inactive in the body and in order to be effective first must be converted to prednisolone by enzymes in the liver. Prednisone may not work as effectively in people with liver disease whose ability to convert prednisone to prednisolone is impaired.

Rayos- Long-acting corticosteroid medication in the form of delayed-release prednisone. This medication releases the action of prednisone about 4 hours after tablets are ingested. Used the treatment of such rheumatoid arthritis polymyalgia rheumatica and also adrenal insufficiency.

## Steroid Equivalent Dose Conversion Chart

| 5mg | 0.8mg | 20mg |
|---|---|---|
| Prednisone | Dexamethasone | Hydrocortisone |

| 4mg | 5mg | 5mg |
|:---:|:---:|:---:|
| MethylPrednisolone | Cortisone | Prednisolone |

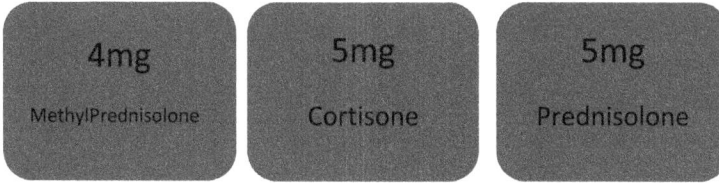

Treatment of Adrenal insufficiency also includes:

- Daily replacement hormone medication(s).
- Proper rest, hydration, stress management and nutrition.
- Knowing the signs of low cortisol (there is currently no meter to check blood levels.)
- Respecting the physical limits of your body.
- Having an emergency injection of cortisol at all times.
- Wearing a medical alert bracelet at all times.

# Chapter 2: Managing Life with Adrenal Insufficiency

The most vital part of managing adrenal insufficiency is arguably the awareness of low cortisol symptoms. Due to the various symptoms, each patient may present with low cortisol in different ways. It is imperative to understand the specific way you or someone you love with adrenal insufficiency presents with low cortisol. Keeping a log of symptoms, daily activities and vital signs is a great way to understand how well adrenal insufficiency is being managed.

**Updosing** is also a vital part of quality of life with adrenal disease. Without sufficient cortisol replacement, an adrenal patient will not have quality of life. Minus what traditional medicine has falsely presented, adrenal disease patients may still severely suffer even on cortisol replacement medications.

The theory behind this is that artificially managing a pulsating hormone exactly the way the human body would is virtually impossible, especially in patients with severe forms of adrenal insufficiency.

All forms of adrenal insufficiency are life threatening but there are variants in the quality of life. Some adrenal patients are able to run marathons and are stable on oral steroid replacement, while others severely struggle with menial tasks such as driving, working and even showering. This is why research and innovation are desperately needed in endocrine medicine. It is not widely understood as to why some adrenal patients struggle more than others.

However, quality of life is the goal with any disease, but specifically with adrenal insufficiency there are many factors that can impact overall wellness. The rest of this chapter will be discussing options that may improve quality of life for adrenal patients.

### Exercise

Exercise can be a difficult task for those with severe forms of adrenal insufficiency. Any extra stressor on the body can be potentially deadly for someone with cortisol deficiency. However, exercise is necessary to prevent muscle wasting and physical deterioration.

Discuss exercise concerns with a physician. You can have a physical evaluation done to assess how receptive your body is to exercise. Once you are physically cleared, you can also try low impact and safe options to lightly introduce your body to more activity. Most insurance policies will cover physical therapy if a doctor deems it medically necessary. Starting a physical therapy regiment with a licensed physical therapist who is trained to work with people with chronic illnesses is a great option.

Find an exercise regimen that does not overwhelm your body. It is also important to give your body the cortisol that it needs to handle the extra physical activity. This may require an increase in your cortisol dose before, during or after your exercise session. Talk with your physician and formulate a plan for updosing for exercise.

## Low Impact Exercise Options

Foam Rolling- A foam roller is a stretching and exercise device created in different sizes and shapes designed to stretch muscles and release tension in targeted muscle areas. This form of exercise is a great, low impact way to gradually build muscle mass. You can do most of these exercises lying down at a slow pace.

Yoga- Yoga is an ancient practice used to increase flexibility, range of motion and relaxation. This exercise, when done slowly can be an easier exercise option for those who struggle to work out due to their health condition. Yoga also incorporates breathing techniques which have been found to reduce stress levels and therefore may reduce your body's stress response.

Swimming- Swimming is a low impact exercise that can build muscular strength and endurance and can improve cardiovascular stamina. You can do this exercise at a slow pace and work your way up to a more intense exercise regimen as your body tolerates.

Sit and be Fit- This fitness series was created in 1987 by Mary Ann Wilson, a registered nurse who specialized in rehabilitation. This series allows people with physical limitations to safely and comfortably exercise. You can find this series online and most libraries carry copies you can rent for free. (You can also find more information at sitandbefit.org)

## Nutrition

Nutrition is a huge part of wellness. What you put in your body is going to have a direct impact on your quality of life. Though no diet can cure adrenal disease, a diet full of vitamins and minerals that avoids sugars and artificial, processed foods is beneficial. Conditions such as insulin resistance and steroid induced diabetes are concerns for those on long-term steroid therapy. Avoiding large amounts of sugar is recommended in those who are on cortisol replacement medications. Processed foods and artificial ingredients may be added metabolic stressors to your body, which are not beneficial to an endocrine system that is already struggling with stress response.

Sodium is also a key dietary component in those with salt wasting forms of adrenal disease. It is important to fulfill salt cravings with healthy options and not always reach for the salty, processed snacks to curb those cravings.

Salt wasting forms of adrenal insufficient diseases may require high sodium diets. Dietary additions such as pickles, Himalayan pink salt and chicken broth may be beneficial.

It is also important to stay hydrated and maintain proper electrolyte homeostasis. Dietary additions of Pedialyte, Gatorade or supplements such as the banana bag powdered solution may be of benefit. (Do not start or stop any electrolyte supplementation without first consulting your healthcare provider.)

Be sure to work with your physician to have frequent lab work to assess your electrolyte levels, which can be abnormal in adrenal disease.

It is also imperative to be aware of your blood glucose, insulin and hemoglobin a1c levels if you are on long term steroid therapy. Your doctor can order these tests to assess your risk of diabetes, which can be increased due to steroids. Eliminating sugary snacks such as soda, cookies, cakes and ice cream can help reduce your risk of developing insulin resistance and type two diabetes. If you do have a sweet tooth, try replacing sugary, processed snacks with healthier options such as raw fruits and natural forms of dark chocolate.
No diet can cure adrenal disease but choosing healthier options can put less stress on the body and may improve your quality of life. Keep a food log of what you eat and how you feel afterwards to assess what diet works best for you. There is currently no standard diet protocol for adrenal insufficiency, only guidelines for healthy eating. Find what works for you.

### Weight

Weight can be a difficult issue with adrenal insufficiency. Most adrenal insufficiency patients suffered unexplained weight loss before diagnosis, only to find themselves at the mercy of the one of most dominant steroid side effects, weight gain. It is important to support your loved one if they are struggling with the physical aspects that long-term steroid use and adrenal disease can cause. It can be an extremely daunting experience to watch a disease transform your body into something you do not even recognize due to no fault of your own. It is important to remind adrenal patients that looks are secondary to quality of life. It is much more important to feel better than it is to look better. Eating the most nutritious diet possible, exercising at a safe and gentle pace and keeping a positive body image are the best treatment options for weight management protocols in adrenal insufficiency.

## Mindset

Mindset is vital to managing any chronic health condition, but especially in the case of adrenal insufficiency. The adrenals are emotionally driven and react to every single emotional situation. The body also reacts to thoughts and the overall mentality it has. If you are constantly in a state of negativity and stress, your body will react to that. Your autonomic nervous system (which is responsible for subconsciously directing functions such as breathing, your heartbeat, and the digestive system) can become overwhelmed and keep you in state of a "Fight or Flight" response. In an adrenal insufficient person, they do not have the luxury of a natural cortisol response. Being in a state of stress is literally detrimental to their health and causes the autonomic nervous system to be on constant alert.

Adrenal insufficiency is a stressful condition as it is and adding other factors such as family issues, raising kids, paying bills and general adult responsibilities can increase your need for cortisol. Therefore, it is vital to have stress management skills and to keep your body out of the "Fight or Flight" state.

To recover from the stressors of life, your body must enter a state of **restorative relaxation**. With a constantly activated autonomic nervous system, your body will not restore itself if it cannot relax.

Though a positive mindset will not cure adrenal disease. However, it may decrease the body's urgency for cortisol and allow you to better manage your adrenal insufficiency.

**Ways to help the body find restorative relaxation:**

1- Affirmations.
It has once been said that perception is reality. Your mind, body and spirit react to the reality they think they are in. If you constantly tell your body it is sick, dying and diseased that is the reality it perceives. When your body thinks it is constantly in danger, it is going to be hyperaware and not enter relaxed state. This is why affirmations are helpful to rewire your brain to perceive a non-threatening reality. Positive affirmations that help your brain escape the "Fight or Flight state" can be as simple as repeating statements such as:

- I am safe. I am okay.
- I can still enjoy life.
- I can find happiness.
- I do *insert enjoyable activity*
- I am worthy of joy, and I will find joy.

2- Meditation.
Whether it is just sitting in silence and focusing on positive thoughts or connecting to nature or praying

to a deity, meditation has been utilized for centuries to induce calmness and restore emotional healing. Daily meditation may help you find more peace of mind and therefore, help you better manage your adrenal disease.

3- Social Support.
Finding supportive people that listen to you and encourage you is a vital part of quality of life. Isolation tends to exacerbate negativity and can be detrimental to those with a scary disease. Reaching out to online support groups, local friends, or community outreaches such as churches and clubs may help you find more peace in your life.

4- Writing/Journaling.
Having a healthy outlet can be beneficial to processing the negative emotions that come with managing a chronic illness. Writing fears, emotions, hopes and dreams down is a
healthy way to express things you may not feel comfortable telling other people. Keeping a daily journal is a great way to release pent up emotions in a healthy way.

5- Purposefully enjoying life.
With a chronic illness, it can be very difficult to keep an attitude of happiness, gratitude and appreciation. When you struggle with things the average person takes for granted, it was a tendency to make the human spirit feel jaded, angry or helpless. Allowing yourself to become a victim to your circumstances will only make matters worse. Life may have dealt you an unfair hand, but it is still your responsibility to play that hand to the best of your abilities. Make it a habit to do something you

enjoy every single day. Whether it is something simple like listening to your favorite music, taking a bubble bath, sitting outside or spending time with loved ones, be sure you are making time for joy in your life.  For every bad thing your health makes you experience, treat yourself to something positive.

6-  Prioritize Self Care.
When bad health days come, it is human nature to get sad, frustrated and overwhelmed when you can't do what you want to do. But in those moments, you can choose to push yourself or you can let your body rest and recover so you can have a better day tomorrow. When your body is already struggling, pushing it when it needs rest is detrimental, especially with adrenal insufficiency. Sometimes you must take the fight lying down. This doesn't make you weak, it makes you smart. With adrenal disease, any stressor on the body is going to tax your cortisol. You do not have the luxury of a properly working adrenal system, so stress is your worst enemy.  Prioritize sleep, relaxation and self-care into your healthcare routine. These things are just as important as food and water!

## Alternative Options

Hormone replacement is the only treatment for adrenal insufficiency. Any vitamin, supplement, diet or treatment that claims to cure adrenal disease is absolutely false. However, there are some treatment additions that many adrenal patients have found benefit from.

In the current atmosphere of people pushing supplements and MLM products to chronically ill people, it is important to discuss any alternative treatment with your physician. Never discontinue your steroids in the hopes that some alternative treatment can replace cortisol. It cannot be done and too many lives have been lost due to steroid withdrawal causing an adrenal crisis. There is no cure for adrenal insufficiency, except in the few cases of recovery from steroid induced secondary adrenal insufficiency.

Adrenal disease patients may be more prone to dehydration, therefore additional fluids such as a saline IV or lactated ringers may be prescribed to help support adrenal patients.

Many herbal supplements claim to be able to impact cortisol levels, so be very wary of these claims. As previously stated, there is no replacement for cortisol other than steroid medication. There is no herb that will successfully sustain the life of someone who is cortisol deficient. Be sure that you mention any herbal treatment to your physician and understand that just because a substance is natural does not mean it does not come with side effects. Do not start or stop any medication, natural remedy, vitamin or herbal supplement without first talking to your healthcare provider.

# Chapter 3: For Family Members/Caregivers/Spouses

The diagnosis of adrenal insufficiency can be a daunting thing for a family member, spouse or loved one to accept. As intimidating as this disease sounds, there is still hope for patients to live a full and happy life.

You, as the caregiver, spouse or loved one, play a major role in the management of adrenal disease. This chapter will discuss the various ways you can help the adrenal insufficient person in your life.

The first step to managing any chronic illness is **understanding**. It is important that you, as part of the support system, understand what form of adrenal disease your loved one has. In the previous chapters, we discussed many forms of adrenal disease. Though they all require cortisol replacement, each form has its own specific challenges. It is also important to understand your loved one's specific health condition. In addition to adrenal disease, are there other conditions, mental health challenges or disabilities they have to manage?

# Basic Necessities

### Steroids

Cortisol replacement medication steroids are essential to life with adrenal disease.
Though they can have a myriad of side effects, steroids cannot be discontinued or adrenal crisis and eventually death will occur without adequate steroid replacement.

**Do not ever suggest your adrenal insufficient loved one discontinue their steroids.**

There is no replacement for cortisol other than steroid medications. No herbal remedy, vitamin, essential oil, exercise, or diet will replace cortisol in the body. Skipping steroid doses is dangerous. Caregivers need to make sure adrenal patients take their steroids.
Suddenly stopping steroids can be life threatening. Do not ever withhold dosing without a doctor's supervision or instruction.

Steroid dosing may differ from day to day depending on the body's physical cortisol needs, which can change in times of stressors such as injury, surgery, pain, emotional situations or grief.

## Sleep

Adrenal insufficiency can be an exhausting disease where fatigue is one of the prominent symptoms. Sleep, proper rest and naps are essential in the life of an adrenal insufficient person.

Do not suggest your loved one "push" through their exhaustion. Respect their limitations. Be understanding that they are not lazy, and this disease can cause low energy levels.

The circadian rhythm is deeply impacted by cortisol, which is one of the most difficult challenges in managing adrenal insufficiency. Cortisol is directly involved in the sleep-wake cycle, and it can be difficult to regulate this cycle with exogenous cortisol replacement medications. One way to regulate this cycle is to make sure your steroid replacement medications are taken according to the circadian rhythm percentages that the body would naturally produce. Cortisol levels are naturally the highest in the morning at the lowest in the evening, with a peak during the early morning hours to help your body achieve wakefulness.

Safe amounts of daily sun exposure is recommended to help regulate the body's circadian rhythm. In addition, avoiding electronics two hours before bedtime and using low lights during the evening such as natural Himalayan salt lamps can help your body regulate the circadian rhythm.

A sleep schedule is also beneficial when you are managing adrenal insufficiency. Improper, non-restorative sleep can cause stress on the body and make the body's need for cortisol increase. It is recommended that adults get at least 7-9 hours of rest.[5]

### Exercise

Adrenal insufficiency patients often struggle with vigorous exercise and extreme fatigue, so exercise may be a struggle for them. Encourage them to do what they can and do not push them past their limits. Suggested low impact exercises are: Walking, swimming, foam rolling or light yoga. Be sure you are supporting your adrenal insufficient loved one and not pushing them past what they are physically able to do. Sometimes, they will have to sit down so they don't fall down and that is okay!

It is important that adrenal patients know that there is a fine line between allowing yourself to be active and pushing your body past what it can do. Never allow your mind to trick you into thinking you can do more than your body will allow. Your brain will lie to you, your body will not.

---

[5] NATIONAL SLEEP FOUNDATION RECOMMENDS NEW SLEEP TIMES | NATIONAL SLEEP FOUNDATION (Sleepfoundation.org, 2015) Sleepfoundation.org. (2015). *National Sleep Foundation Recommends New Sleep Times | National Sleep Foundation*. [online] Available at: https://www.sleepfoundation.org/press-release/national-sleep-foundation-recommends-new-sleep-times

# Emotional Wellbeing

Understand that adrenal disease can affect physical abilities, appearance, weight, careers, mental health, finances, relationships and self-esteem. Be kind, be supportive and understanding with your loved one suffering from adrenal disease. Accept them for who they are now and help them deal with the changes caused by this disease.

Also understand that low cortisol can present with mental health changes such as crying, anger, anxiety and depression. If your loved one is experiencing any of these symptoms, please ensure they have adequate amounts of cortisol replacement and remind them to updose as needed.

Panic attacks, night terrors and an overall feeling of anxiety have been widely expressed by adrenal patients as a possible symptom of low cortisol. It is important to keep feelings of anxiety and panic under control with adrenal disease, as these feelings can increase the body's need for cortisol. Changes in mental health status need to be addressed by a healthcare provider as soon as they occur. Adrenal patients' cortisol needs may be directly impacted by their emotions. Any stress on the body, even positive stress can cause an increased need for cortisol. A normal functioning adrenal gland will release cortisol in response to emotional or physical stress, an adrenal insufficient person's body will not.

# Diet

Adrenal insufficiency patients may require high sodium diets to manage salt wasting forms of this disease. Dietary additions such as pickles, Himalayan pink salt and chicken broth may be beneficial. It is also important to stay hydrated and maintain proper electrolyte homeostasis. Dietary additions of Pedialyte, Gatorade or supplements such as the banana bag solution may be of benefit. (Do not start or stop any electrolyte supplementation without first consulting your healthcare provider.)

## Stress Management

Stress can harm an adrenal insufficient person. Arguments, tension, sadness, fear, anger and grief can require an increase in the body's need for cortisol. Remind your loved one to updose in times of physical and emotional stress. Understand that both "good" and "bad" stress can require more cortisol.

Cortisol needs can change from day to day depending on physical or emotional stressors. It is important to have adequate cortisol replacement daily. Adrenal patients need to updose their steroid if they are feeling symptoms of low cortisol. It is important to updose beforehand if they know they are entering a situation that will require more cortisol. Adrenal disease requires adequate steroid replacement, proper hydration, healthy nutrition and stress management. Support from family members and friends can benefit the lives of adrenal patients.

# Adrenal Crisis

(This information is not meant to replace medical care. Please discuss adrenal crisis symptoms and treatment with an endocrinologist.)

An adrenal crisis[6] is defined as a life- threatening, medical emergency caused by insufficient levels of the hormone,

---

[6] ACUTE ADRENAL CRISIS - (ADDISONIAN CRISIS)
In-text: (Uclahealth.org, n.d.): Uclahealth.org. (n.d.). Acute Adrenal Crisis - (Addisonian crisis). [online] Available at:

cortisol. It will lead to certain death if left untreated and must be quickly addressed to prevent organ and nervous system damage.

An adrenal crisis can be caused by any physical or emotional stressor that exceeds the amount of cortisol the adrenal patient has in their body from their steroid medication. Since adrenal patients cannot make their own cortisol, if a situation drains more than their steroid provides, they will need extra steroid medication to cope with the stress.

## Possible Adrenal Crisis Symptoms[7]

This is not an all-inclusive list. Every adrenal patient may present with different crisis symptoms. It is important to discuss symptoms with your adrenal disease patient to understand their specific symptoms of low cortisol.

- Changes in Mental Status
- Changes in Heart Rate
- Changes in Blood Pressure
- Flank pain
- Loss of consciousness
- Dehydration
- Dizziness or lightheadedness
- Fatigue
- Weakness

---

https://www.uclahealth.org/endocrine-center/acute-adrenal-crisis.

[7] KIRKLAND, MD, FACP, FCCM, MSHA, L.
Adrenal Crisis: Background, Pathophysiology, Epidemiology
In-text: (Kirkland, MD, FACP, FCCM, MSHA, 2018: Kirkland, MD, FACP, FCCM, MSHA, L. (2018). Adrenal Crisis: Background, Pathophysiology, Epidemiology. [online] Emedicine.medscape.com. Available at: https://emedicine.medscape.com/article/116716-overview.

- Headache
- Vomiting
- Nausea

**Possible Causes of Adrenal Crisis**

- Physical stressors on the body such as pain, surgery, vomiting, exercise, hunger, exposure to extreme temperatures, hunger, dehydration or allergic reactions.
- Emotional stressors such as traumatic experiences, death of a loved one, sudden shock/surprise, arguments, or tense situations.
- Car accidents, injuries or any physical trauma.
- Certain medications can impact the absorption of oral steroid medications and can cause adrenal crisis if there is a severe drug interaction.

### Treating an Adrenal Crisis

- Give an emergency steroid injection to an adrenal patient showing crisis symptoms or if they are unconscious.
- Call 911
- Recommended emergency department care is to administer steroids to stabilize the adrenal disease patient. Cortisol is imperative to sustaining life in adrenal insufficient patients.
- Withholding a steroid injection during a crisis may result in organ damage and if left untreated, adrenal crisis will result in death.
- Administering a steroid injection is imperative to successfully treating an adrenal crisis.

In the event of an adrenal crisis, a steroid injection **must** be administered. Do not ever hesitate to inject an adrenal insufficient patient with solu-cortef.

### How to Administer Solu-Cortef Acto-Vial Emergency Cortisol Injection

1. Remove the two-chamber vial containing Solu-Cortef Act-O-Vial from the packaging.
   a. Press the colored cap down to mix solvent with the powder solution of hydrocortisone.
   b. Mix the contents until the powder is completed dissolved. The powder solution of hydrocortisone is completely dissolved once the solution is clear.
2. Remove the protective disc from the center of the plastic cap of the vial.
3. Wipe top of vial with alcohol swab to sterilize it before inserting syringe into bottle.
4. Insert the syringe into the vial. Turn the vial upside down and draw the solution into the syringe.
5. Hold the syringe like a dart and push the needle for 2/3 of its length into the chosen injection site at a right angle to the skin.
6. Give the injection into intramuscular tissue such as the buttock or in the upper thigh muscle.

# Emergency Medical Service Protocols

Emergency Management Services (EMS) protocols can differ according to the country you live in. In the United States, each state's counties may have different legislation regarding the administration of Solu-Cortef. EMS may be organized by the city services, by the county itself, or independently owned by private companies. According to how they operate, they may or may not have established protocols on how to treat an adrenal crisis. You can find out if adrenal insufficiency protocols are in place by visiting your local station, calling the county for information and/or contacting EMS director or fire chief. You may also want to check online on your local county website to see if specific protocols are posted.

If the website provides a searchable document format look for the following phrases:
- Solu-cortef, solucortef, cortef
- Solu-medrol, solumedrol
- Adrenal crisis, acute adrenal

Find a point of contact to submit your protocol questions regarding the administration of Solu-Cortef.

Keep respect and professionalism in mind when corresponding and making requests. You may mention you are a volunteer with Adrenal Alternatives Foundation and provide them with our contact information if you wish.

Possible Points of Contact:
- Fire Chief
- EMS Director
- Training Development Coordinator
- Medical Director

Present a well-formed case to your point of contact. You can provide them with pamphlets on how to properly treat an adrenal crisis. It is important to have both factual and humanitarian aspects in your correspondence with your point of contact. Solu-Cortef administration can be the difference in life or death in adrenal insufficient patients. Be sure you are making that point very clear in your intentions to update EMS protocols. If your current county does not allow the administration of Solu-Cortef, provide them with the necessary information on how you would like to see this protocol added.

Suggested Protocol Addendums for the treatment of an Adrenal Crisis:
- Allow paramedics/EMT staff to administer patient carried Solu-Cortef medications.
- Provide training to all EMS personnel via educational handouts, videos or seminar education.
- Many organizations such as Adrenal Alternatives Foundation have pre-made information you can present to your local EMS providers.

# Chapter 4: Critical Care

### Patient Perspective VS Outdated Research

Upon working with the adrenal disease demographic with the Adrenal Alternatives Foundation, a consistent message our patients tend to relate is that they feel their endocrinologists or physicians do not understand the full gravity of the toll this disease takes on quality of life. According to the textbooks, with adrenal insufficiency, a person should be able to take a steroid tablet a few times a day and resume a normal life. For those with severe forms of adrenal disease, nothing could be further from the truth.

This is why much research is desperately needed to discover why some patents struggle so heavily with quality of life and complain of symptoms that they are told are "unrelated" to adrenal insufficiency.

From a patient perspective, having watched thousands of adrenal insufficient patients suffer with this disease, it is our hope that this book provides a new insight into the reality of life with adrenal insufficiency. It is also our goal that this narrative inspires more conversations on how we can find better treatment protocols and research improvements to improve quality of life.

The standard treatment protocols have not changed since Thomas Addison was the first to describe adrenal failure in 1855. Modern endocrinology teaches that steroid tablets given two to three times daily is an adequate enough treatment to manage the pulsating hormone, glucocorticoid hormone, cortisol.

With adrenal insufficiency, a person is not only replacing a missing hormone(s), but also trying to replicate a major body system. In a normal adrenal gland, it will produce various amounts of cortisol in accordance to the stressors it is exposed to. In an adrenal insufficient patient, this must be artificially done. With the newer research on the importance of circadian rhythm[8] dosing, adrenal patients are now seeking a better way to replace their cortisol.

Adrenal patients with other health issues or diseases, especially conditions which cause chronic pain and comorbidities that impact the absorption of oral steroid tablets tend not to be as stable as those who only have the single diagnosis of adrenal insufficiency.

---

[8] CHAN, D. S. AND DEBONO, M.
Replication of cortisol circadian rhythm: new advances in hydrocortisone replacement therapy Chan, D. and Debono, M.Therapeutic Advances in Endocrinology and Metabolism. Available at: https://www.ncbi.nlm.nih.gov/pmc/articles/PMC3475279/.

Which begs the question, is there really a "standard" dose for cortisol?

In the Adrenal Alternatives Foundation's research[9], we have found that the answer is no. With the cortisol pumping survey, we asked anonymous adrenal insufficient patients questions regarding their quality of life pre- and post-pump therapy.

Below are the answers participants stated when asked what their average basal dose of solu-cortef was:

| 40mg | 25mg | 27mg | 50.75mg | 23.65mg | 46mg | 18.75mg | 22.8mg | 22.49mg | 42mg |
|------|------|------|---------|---------|------|---------|--------|---------|------|
| 20mg | 41.8mg | 34mg | 35mg | 38mg | 32.6mg | 36 mg | 44.4mg | 23.5 | 32mg |
| 45mg | 27.5mg | 21.3mg | 43mg | 62.5mg | 28.4mg | 39.6mg | 29.7 | 30mg | 10mg |
| 39mg | 25mg | 35mg | 30mg | 45mg | 30mg | 24mg | 60mg | 24mg | 25mg |

As you can see, the dosing widely varies. This is why treatment for adrenal insufficiency must be individualized and based off of quality of life and not a standard dose. Physical, lifestyle and emotional stressors can impact the body's need for cortisol and that is one reason why cortisol deficiency can be so difficult to treat.

It is the hope of the Adrenal Alternatives Foundation that we can educate the medical community on the reality of how this disease truly is. It is not as simple as replacing cortisol, it involves a myriad of regulation to find quality of life in some patients.

One of the greatest fears of many adrenal insufficient patients is how cortisol deficiency is a relatively unknown

---

[9] CORTISOL PUMPING SURVEY (adrenalalternatives.com, 2020): adrenalalternatives.com. (2020). Cortisol Pumping Survey. [online] Available at: https://docs.google.com/forms/d/1eWYZjIFP9HRJDosvdimJnOr8p54R mpx_2A4Xz40f77A/edit#responses.

issue in the emergency medical system. As previously stated, most emergency medical services are not legally allowed to administer solu-cortef and it is not a standard medication carried on most ambulances. To make matters worse, emergency room physicians can be unwilling to administer steroids. Many unfortunate deaths have happened within the adrenal community due to this negligence. Far too many lives have been lost simply due to the withholding of steroid medications. Steroids save lives and are a necessary intervention in the treatment of an adrenal crisis. Organ damage and eventual death will occur if cortisol is not administered in an appropriate time period in someone with adrenal insufficiency. Not to mention an adrenal crisis is a severely terrifying and painful event that can cause damage to the body and impair quality of life.

## Emergency Room Guidelines

One of the trickiest parts of adrenal insufficiency is that not everyone presents with an adrenal crisis in the same manner. Emergency room healthcare providers may confuse an adrenal crisis with other issues such as anxiety attacks, allergic reactions, psychiatric breakdowns or even gastrointestinal sickness.

It is imperative that steroids be administered to someone presenting with abnormal symptoms outside of their baseline if they have a diagnosis of adrenal insufficiency.

The standard protocol for treating an adrenal crisis[10] is the administration of an intravenous steroid or intramuscular injection of solu-cortef. Supportive treatment of

---

[10] ACUTE ADRENAL CRISIS - (ADDISONIAN CRISIS: (Uclahealth.org. (n.d.). Acute Adrenal Crisis - (Addisonian crisis). [online] Available at: https://www.uclahealth.org/endocrine-center/acute-adrenal-crisis

intravenous fluids is usually accompanied with continued monitoring of vital signs and improvement of symptoms. What cortisol the body does not use will excrete through the urine so overdose from an emergency injection is virtually impossible. Too much cortisol will not cause death, too little will. Withholding of steroid medications to an adrenal insufficient patient is not only life-threatening but arguably inhumane.

**An adrenal crisis will result in death if left untreated**.

With this knowledge, it is our hope that emergency room healthcare providers do not hesitate to provide the necessary lifesaving interventions to treat an adrenal crisis in a timely manner.

## Surgical Guidelines

During a surgical procedure, the body will require an increase in steroid dosing. Surgery is one of the most prominent activators of the HPA axis. Researchers[11] have reported HPA axis function during and after surgical procedures that plasma cortisol levels increase significantly. In patients without the presence of adrenal insufficiency, cortisol production rates increased to 75–150 mg/day after major surgery.

---

[11] JUNG, C. AND INDER, W. J.
Management of adrenal insufficiency during the stress of medical illness and surgery: Jung, C. and Inder, W. (2008). Management of adrenal insufficiency during the stress of medical illness and surgery. [online] Australasian Medical Publishing Company. Available at: https://www.mja.com.au/journal/2008/188/7/management-adrenal-insufficiency-during-stress-medical-illness-and-surgery .

In adrenal insufficient patients, the recommendations differ deepening on the length and severity of the procedure being performed. It is important to note that adrenal insufficiency patients will always require additional glucocorticoid supplementation during surgery, but there is no uniform standard accepted regimen for glucocorticoid replacement therapy. It is the best clinical practice to treat the patient instead of following a textbook response. If a patient with adrenal insufficiency is declining, the administration of more cortisol should be a first line treatment protocol.

However, there are suggested recommendations: [12]

**For Minor Surgery:** Double or triple the usual daily dose of glucocorticoid until recovery. Intravenous hydrocortisone 25 mg or equivalent at start of procedure. Usual replacement dose after procedure.

**For Dental Procedures:** Under local anesthesia, double the daily dose of glucocorticoid on the day of procedure. Inject 100mg emergency cortisol injection if patient presents with adrenal crisis symptoms.

**For Moderate Surgery:** Intravenous hydrocortisone 75 mg/day on day of procedure (25 mg 8-hourly). Intravenous hydrocortisone 25 mg 8-hourly until recovery. Taper over next 1–2 days to usual replacement dose in uncomplicated cases.

---

[12] COLLARD MD, C. D., SAATEE, M.D, S., REIDY, M.D, A. B. AND LIU, M.D, M. M. Perioperative Steroid Management: Approaches Based on Current Evidence: Collard MD, C., Saatee, M.D, S., Reidy, M.D, A. and Liu, M.D, M. (2017). Perioperative Steroid Management: Approaches Based on Current Evidence. [online] Anesthesiology: Trusted Evidence Discovery in Practice. Available at: https://anesthesiology.pubs.asahq.org/article.aspx?articleid=2626031

**For Major Surgery:**
Intravenous hydrocortisone 150 mg/day (50 mg 8-hourly)
Taper over next 2–3 days only once clinical condition
stabilizes.

**For critical illness/intensive care/major trauma or life-threatening complications:**
200 mg/day intravenous hydrocortisone (50 mg 6-hourly,
or by continuous infusion)

**Note:** There is no universally agreed upon standard dose or
duration of exogenous steroids used to treat adrenal
insufficiency. Clinicians must be observant of a patient's
vital signs, empirical evidence and quality of life. It is also
imperative clinicians be aware of the symptoms of adrenal
crisis, which can widely vary in patients. In the event these
symptoms should arise, an immediate dose of
glucocorticoids should be administered until patient
stabilizes.

# Chapter 5:
# Cortisol Pumping Method

### Subcutaneous Cortisol Injections [13]

There are "alternative" treatment options that not many
endocrinologists are aware of. In patients who have poor
absorption due to gastrointestinal problems or have
comorbid issues that prevent their ability to metabolize oral

---

[13] SUBCUTANEOUS HYDROCORTISONE ADMINISTRATION
FOR EMERGENCY USE IN ADRENAL INSUFFICIENCY. -
PUBMED – NCBI: Ncbi.nlm.nih.gov. (2013). Subcutaneous
hydrocortisone administration for emergency use in adrenal
insufficiency. - PubMed - NCBI. [online] Available at:
https://www.ncbi.nlm.nih.gov/pubmed/23672956.

steroids may find benefit from using multiple daily injections of cortisol or by using an infusion pump. These concepts are very similar to how diabetic patients use insulin, only in adrenal insufficiency patients, they are using cortisol (Solu-Cortef) instead.

With these treatment options, patients calculate their current oral steroid dose to a 1:1 or 2:1 ratio.

1:1 Ratio is 1ML of saline per 100mg Solu-Cortef. 1 unit=1mg.

2:1 Ratio is 2ML of saline per 100mg Solu Cortef. 2units = 2mg.

To start subQ injections, an adrenal patient will need to convert their current oral steroid dose amount and set an injection schedule to administer the cortisol according to their personal cortisol clearance rate and also by circadian rhythm dosing percentages. It is important to note that with cortisol replacement, the right time the medication is given is just as important as the right dose. It is completely possible to be both over and under replaced in the same day. This is why cortisol clearance testing is a great tool to assess how effective replacement therapy is in adrenal insufficiency.

## Example Case Study

Jane is a 32-year-old female who was diagnosed with adrenal insufficiency after presenting to the emergency department with low blood pressure, recent unexplained weight loss and hyperpigmentation. Jane had a previous diagnosis of Crohn's disease and attributed all her new symptoms to that diagnosis, to which her physician disagreed with and suspected adrenal disease. Upon a cortisol lab draw, her results came back alarmingly low. She was then immediately referred to an endocrinologist and an ATCH stimulation test was immediately performed. Jane's results confirmed the diagnosis of adrenal insufficiency. She was then placed on oral hydrocortisone tablets. Initially she stabilized but then continued to decline in her health. Her frequent vomiting and gastrointestinal symptoms due to the Crohn's disease made her compliance to oral steroid replacement difficult. She voiced her concerns to her physician, who suggested she try subcutaneous injections of cortisol instead of oral tablets.

**Jane's Dosing schedule on tablets**:
6am- 15mg
9am-10mg
2pm- 5mg
6pm-5mg
9pm-2.5mg
Total: 37.5mg

**Jane's Dosing schedule calculated on SubQ Injections**:
(1:1 Ratio is 1ML of saline per 100mg Solu-cortef)
3am- 10units
6am-15units
11am- 5units
4pm-5units
7pm-2.5units
Total: 37.5 units

Subcutaneous injections may be a viable option for those who are not stabilized on oral steroids or who are waiting to begin the cortisol pumping method. This treatment option bypasses the oral/stomach route and may be especially beneficial to those who suffer from malabsorption and are hyper-metabolizers.

## How to start Subcutaneous Cortisol Injections

- Discuss this treatment option with your physician. You will need them to write a prescription for Solu-Cortef, which is the powdered version of cortisol.
- Solu-Cortef comes in two options:

1-Solu-Cortef Powder Vials
2- Actovials, which contain 2ML of saline.

You and your physician can decide which ratio is best for you.

- You will also need the following supplies: Alcohol prep pads, Needles, Saline or Bacteriostatic water.
- Choose your medication ratio (1:1 or 2:1)
- Work with your physician to calculate your injection schedule.
- To figure out your baseline dose, convert oral milligrams you are currently taking in tablets from to solu-cortef units.

Be sure you are cleaning the area with alcohol before you inject. Also note that saline and bacteriostatic water must be refrigerated once they have been opened.

## Subcutaneous Cortisol Injection Protocol

1- Clean the top of the saline or bacteriostatic water with an alcohol prep.
2- Place a sterile needle into the saline or bacteriostatic water vial and draw 1ML if you are doing 1:1 ratio or draw 2ML if you are doing 2:2 ratio.
3- Inject the bacteriostatic water or saline into the vial of Solu-Cortef powder.
4- Shake until the mixture is clear.

5- Prep your injection with an alcohol wipe.
6- Draw your dose into a sterile needle or insulin syringe.
7- Inject into fatty tissue. (Thighs, abdomen, back of arms, etc.)
8- Be sure to rotate injection sites.

**What is the Cortisol Pump?**

Adrenal Insufficiency and Diabetes are both difficult diseases to manage. Both are serious, endocrine disorders. Adrenal insufficiency is a disease where the adrenal glands fail to produce the proper amounts of steroid hormones. There are many different forms of adrenal disease, but the treatment for all forms is the same- steroids for cortisol replacement. Type 1 Diabetes is the disease where the pancreas fails to produce the correct amount of insulin, thus rendering someone insulin dependent. Both of these diseases are endocrine disorders. Both of these diseases require life-long replacement therapy. The adrenal insufficient person is dependent on cortisol. The diabetic is dependent on insulin. Both of these diseases are life threatening. Both of these diseases require daily monitoring.

Almost every cell in the body has cortisol receptors, making it a crucial hormone. This hormone impacts multiple functions of the body. Without adequate levels of cortisol, the body will go into an adrenal crisis which will result in organ failure and eventually death. Cortisol impacts blood sugar levels, metabolism, stress response, inflammation levels, aids in the immune system, affects the metabolic processes such as the salt and water balances within the body and it also greatly impacts the circadian rhythm.

Unlike diabetic patients, adrenal disease sufferers have no meter to check their cortisol levels. They must be constantly vigilant of their own personal signs and symptoms of low cortisol and require an emergency injection if their levels drop too low. The standard treatment for all adrenal disease patients is daily cortisol replacement medication- steroids.

Medications such as prednisone, dexamethasone or hydrocortisone are prescribed to replace the deficits of steroid hormones in the body. Steroids have a myriad of side effects ranging from weight gain to emotional disturbances. Long term steroid use has been linked to damage to the bones, eyesight and even muscle tissue. Yet, steroid hormone replacement is the only treatment for adrenal disease. In a normal person, during situations of emotional or physical stress their body releases more cortisol. The excitement from a happy event, the sadness from a death of a loved one or the strain from exercising are examples of things that would cause the body to release more cortisol. In an adrenal insufficient person, this does not happen. They must artificially manage their cortisol. Their personal cortisol needs may differ from day to day. No two days are the same and it is a struggle to regulate proper cortisol levels.

The most commonly prescribed steroid for adrenal insufficiency is hydrocortisone (HC). This is the bio-identical steroid medication. This medication has a blood serum half-life of 90 minutes and must be taken multiple times a day. Many adrenal patients struggle with quality of life due to this mismanagement. Oral HC must be processed through the stomach and the liver before reaching the blood stream. This causes a rise and fall of cortisol levels, which can result in subpar function, can increase mortality rates and can decrease quality of life.

Quality of life in adrenal disease patients can be vastly poor due to this lack of balance. Oral cortisol replacement cannot do what natural cortisol can. But fortunately, endocrinology research has found a solution for adrenal patients who have failed to stabilize on oral cortisol replacement medications. The concept of Cortisol Pumping is the use of solu-cortef (inject-able version of cortisol) mixed with saline or bacteriostatic water used in an insulin pump programmed to disperse cortisol according to the natural circadian rhythm by programming rates of delivery into the pump. This therapy bypasses the gastric passage and is able to deliver cortisol in a more natural way. With this method, an adrenal insufficient patient can receive a constant supply of cortisol and will not suffer the instability experienced with oral steroid cortisol replacement. Side effects due to malabsorption are decreased and patients have been reported to have improved sleep, weight management and experience an overall improvement in their energy levels and sense of well-being. This method has also been proven to lessen the prevalence of adrenal crises and lessen hospitalizations due to low cortisol.

Though this method is not a cure for adrenal disease, it is an option and a ray of hope for those who are struggling with quality of life.

According to a survey done by the Adrenal Alternatives Foundation[14] concluded that 94.2% of the 52 anonymous cortisol pumping patients reported that the cortisol pump had improved their quality of life.

---

[14] CORTISOL PUMPING SURVEY
adrenalalternatives.com. (2020). Cortisol Pumping Survey. [online] Available at:
https://docs.google.com/forms/d/1eWYZjIFP9HRJDosvdimJnOr8p54R
mpx_2A4Xz40f77A/edit#responses

Has it improved your quality of life?

52 responses

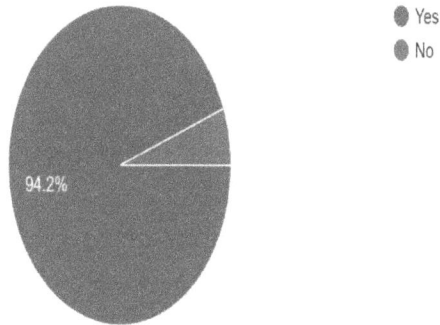

94.2%

● Yes
● No

## Disclaimers:

Every adrenal patient is different and there is no "normal" dose for cortisol pumping.

The cortisol pumping method is not a cure for adrenal insufficiency and is not a "plug in and fix" treatment. Adrenal insufficiency is life threatening and must be properly treated.

The cortisol pumping method is not a replacement for an emergency cortisol injection.

### How to Start the Cortisol Pumping Method

1- Assess your life, health and disease management.

The cortisol pump is not a cure for adrenal insufficiency and is not a treatment that is right for everyone. If you are well managed on the steroid replacement pills, the adrenal pump is excess money and effort you may not need. The pump is not an easy thing to acquire and the fight to get one takes a great deal of trouble, mental stamina and resources.

2- Research, learn and educate for yourself.

Information you need to know:

- What form of adrenal insufficiency do you have?

- What is your quality of life?

- Are you able to work, drive, do housework or function normally?

- What have you tried to manage your adrenal disease?

- What is your current daily dose of replacement steroid?

- How much are you stress dosing?

- What other medical issues do you have?

- Are you able to afford the supplies and medication needed for the pump?

(Insurance may or may not cover your pump, supplies or solu-cortef.)

3- Find a Pump Friendly Physician.

Prepare the best case possible. Send your research, your health information and everything you can to the physician before your appointment, so they are aware of your intentions beforehand. You can also write a letter to the physician explaining your diagnosis, failed treatments and desire to be on the pump. There is a letter template on the Adrenal Alternatives Foundation website (https://adrenalalternatives.com/downloadable-materials/) that you can fill out with your information and send to your physician before your appointment. Keep in mind this treatment is a nuance and they may or may not be receptive to your request. Therefore, sending a letter beforehand informing them of your intentions may save you time, money and effort.  You may have to query multiple physicians before you find one who is willing to manage your care on the pump.

4- Battling the Insurance Company.

Adrenal Insufficiency is documented to be treated by oral steroids and not by the infusion pump method but there are options to attempt insurance coverage for the use of infusion pumps in adrenal disease.

### Cortisol Pumping Basics

1– Find the right pump system.

There are multiple different pump systems available. Determining what company works best for you will depend on your personal cortisol needs, what your insurance will cover and your lifestyle. Though the concept of all pumps is the same, some have different features such as being waterproof or tubeless.

2– Choosing a Solu-Cortef ratio.

Solu-Cortef comes in two forms, Acto-Vials and powder vials. The actovials are Solu-Cortef powder that is attached with 2ML of saline solution at the top of the canister. The powder vials are only Solu-Cortef.

With Acto-vials, the ratio is 2:1. This means that 2ml of solution is equal to 2mg of cortisol because 100mg of solu-cortef was mixed with the 2ml of saline contained in the canister and reconstituted before adding it into the pump reservoir. Pump distribution rates will be calculated according to this.

Example-If a patient takes 20 mg daily their basal rate will be 40units.

2units= 2mg at the 2:1 ratio.

With the powder solu-cortef vials, patients can run a 1:1 ratio by mixing the 100mg of Solu-Cortef powder with 1ML of saline or bacteriostatic water and reconstituting it with a syringe before adding it into the pump reservoir.

Example-If a patient takes 35 mg daily, their basal rate will be 35units. 1unit= 1mg at the 1:1 ratio.

 3– Finding the right basal dose and rate distribution. Cortisol replacement therapy needs to be a personalized, calculated process where many things are considered.

A– Your personal absorption. Clearance testing labs can be done to determine how quickly your body metabolizes cortisol.

B– Your daily basal dose needs. Every adrenal patient is different. Your dose will depend on your specific body's needs according to your health status, comorbidities, pain levels, weight, and cortisol clearance.

C– Your distribution rates. Cortisol replacement needs to be done as closely to the circadian rhythm as possible. 24-hour profiles can be done to try and match your body's natural process of cortisol production.

 4– Managing "artificial adrenals."
The pump truly puts adrenal patients in control of their cortisol distribution in a way that steroid pills cannot. In situations of physical or emotional stress where "updosing" is needed, the pump can immediately administer a bolus, which is extra cortisol administered through the pump canula at the amount you select. Instead of having to wait 30-90 minutes for pills to metabolize, the cortisol can be absorbed faster and may be able to better help prevent an adrenal crisis.

5- Supplies needed:
- Alcohol Prep Pads
- Infusion Pump
- Infusion Sets
- Saline or Bacteriostatic Water
- Solu-Cortef
- Syringes
- Sharps Container

Additionally helpful supplies:
- Band-Aids
- Hibiclens solution
- Medical paper tape
- Skin Tac
- Tegaderms

- Label stating your pump is cortisol and not insulin.

## Pre-Pump Lab Assessments

It is important to note that the cortisol pump is only as effective as the information programmed into it, which is why proper evaluation and testing is necessary for the effectiveness of this treatment. As previously mentioned, there are many factors which will determine an adrenal insufficient patient's cortisol needs.

Cortisol clearance testing is vital to the success of the cortisol pumping method. It is important to evaluate how quickly an adrenal insufficient person's body sustains cortisol in their system. Dosing needs to be calculated specifically to how fast a person's body metabolizes cortisol. This can be assessed by completing a cortisol day curve test. The test measures your blood cortisol levels every hour for 24 hours.

## Establishing a Pumping Care Plan

Creating a successful care plan with the cortisol pumping method is reliant on a variety of factors. As previously mentioned, cortisol clearance needs to be evaluated first. Once that has been completed, it is important to use that information to formulate appropriate distribution rates that can be programmed into the infusion pump.

Rates need to be calculated according to the results of the cortisol clearance testing, circadian rhythm percentages, empirical patient symptoms and overall wellness. The body naturally produces cortisol at different intervals throughout the day, the highest being in the morning to generate the natural waking response and the lowest in the evening to induce sleep. Cortisol levels will also rise in accordance to stressors such as exercise, pain or emotional situations. All these factors must be considered when programming an infusion pump for cortisol distribution.

Patients need to work with their physicians to calculate the best possible care plan for quality of life. It is vital to keep track of blood pressure, heart rate, overall feeling of wellness, low cortisol symptoms, stress tolerance, energy levels and physical stamina. Every adrenal patient is different and steroid replacement needs to be tailored to each patient depending on their health status and lifestyle. Steroids can cause side effects and the right dosing at the right time is imperative to achieve quality of life. Steroid dosing may differ from day to day depending on the body's physical cortisol needs, which can change in times of stressors such as injury, surgery, pain, emotional situations or grief.

Replacement needs may differ from day to day depending on the stressors the body may be exposed to. It is not only important to establish a basal rate but also to create a plan for updosing or bolusing for times when extra cortisol is needed. The amount of extra cortisol needed will depend on personal cortisol clearance and the body's stress tolerance. Adrenal patients may exhibit low cortisol in various symptoms. It is vital to know your own personal signs and symptoms of low cortisol and updose at the first symptom. Playing cortisol catch up is a dangerous game that no adrenal patient needs to play.

**Cortisol Care Plan Basics:**

- Daily Basal Rates
- Rates for Sickness/Activity/Etc.
- Temp Basal Rates for Updosing

- Solu-Cortef Ratio (1:1 or 2:1)

**Bolusing/Updosing Protocols:**

- Exercise
- Emotional Stress (Grief, Trauma, etc.)
- Physical Exertion (Household tasks, etc.)
- Emergency Situations (Accidents, etc.)
- Surgery
- Sickness (Fever, Vomiting, etc.)
- Pain
- Extreme Temperatures (Heat or Cold)

Physicians can also repeat the 24-hour cortisol day curve testing to evaluate the efficacy of the cortisol replacement after a patient begins the infusion pumping method. However, it must be stressed that quality of life should be the standard by which the efficacy of the cortisol pumping method is judged. If a patient is still suffering with low cortisol symptoms, the pump rates should be re-evaluated despite lab work being within a normal range.

## Life with the Cortisol Pump

### Showering

Depending on what pump system you have, showering may be a challenge. If you have a non-waterproof tubed system, you will need to pause your cortisol distribution and disconnect from your pump to shower. You can also plan your shower days around your site changes or simply disconnect from the pump and cover your site with a tegaderm and reconnect after your shower.

If you have a tubed waterproof pump however, you can shower with it by using a waist or arm band to keep it in place. There are also completely waterproof and tubeless pumps where showering is completely uninhibited.

**Traveling**

Traveling with the pump through airports, train or bus stations is much easier with preparation and documentation. It is a good idea to have documentation written from your doctor of your diagnosis, what to do for emergency protocols and the necessity of your pump. Most travel companies and airlines will allow you to call ahead and request disability services and you may even have baggage fees waived if luggage contains medical equipment. Be sure you are traveling with proper documentation and your supplies are organized. Always have more than enough supplies for the length of your stay and label everything with your name, diagnosis and treatment protocols. Planning ahead can make a major difference in the ease and success of your travels with the cortisol pump. You may also want to consider bringing a backup pump or subcutaneous injection supplies in case your pump fails during your travels. It is not recommended that certain pumps go through the machines at the airport, so you can request a hand check with TSA instead. Not all pumps need this precaution. Be sure to research the specifics of the pump system you are traveling with.

**Wearing the Pump**

Each pump system is different, some are bulkier than others and have tubing, while others can be easily hidden. Be sure you are placing your sites in areas that have optimal absorption and your clothes are loose enough to prevent occlusions. You can utilize arm bands and belts to clamp your pump to if you are using a tubed system, or simply clip it to your clothing.

## Site Preparation and Removal

It is important to have proper site hygiene to prevent infection. However, the skin's microbiome is sensitive, and it is important to remove sites if they are showing signs of irritation. There are many products you can use pre and post site change such as alcohol swabs, hibiclens, and aloe adhesive remover wipes. Topical creams such as Neosporin or colloidal silver can also be used to help sites heal. Consult with your physician for the best recommendations for your site care. Please also consult your physician if you are showing any signs of infection such as elevated body temperature and sites that are tender, red and hot to the touch.

## Site Changes:

1. Cleanse the top of a saline or bacteriostatic water vial.
2. Fill a sterile syringe with 1 or 2 ML of saline or bacteriostatic water depending on the cortisol ratio you and your doctor chose. (1ml = 1:1 ratio or 2ml = 2:1 ratio)
3. Fill the Solu-Cortef vial with saline or bacteriostatic water.
4. Shake until solution is clear.
5. Fill your pump reservoir with the Solu-Cortef solution. (Note: Different pumps may hold more Solu-Cortef than others.)
6. Prime your pump to be ready to distribute the medication. (Each pump system requires different settings, work with your local pump representative for training if you have questions.)

7. Cleanse your chosen site area. Choose a site with unbroken, subcutaneous tissue.
8. Apply your site and watch for signs of low cortisol. (Note: If your site is not properly absorbing, you will need to change it immediately when you notice low cortisol symptoms.)
9. Be sure the pump is distributing properly, and all alarms and notifications are set to where you can hear the alerts.
10. If in doubt, always change the site if you feel low cortisol symptoms!

Reminder, the cortisol pump is NOT a replacement for an emergency cortisol injection.

# Chapter 6: Miscellaneous Care Concerns

### Blood Donation

Donating blood is one of the most selfless acts a person can do, but when you have a life-threatening illness such as adrenal insufficiency, there are questions as to whether you are allowed to donate blood or not.

Can adrenal disease patients donate blood? The answer is complicated. Some countries/territories allow blood donation from adrenal patients and others do not. It is ultimately dependent on the medical director's decision of a particular organization.

According to the Pituitary Foundation[15], Addison's disease is listed as a permanent deferral which means those with this diagnosis are permanently banned from donating blood.

The Joint United Kingdom (UK) Blood Transfusion and Tissue Transplantation Services Professional Advisory Committee [16]states that anyone diagnosed with any form of adrenal failure "Must not donate."

The American Red Cross [17]website contained no information regarding eligibility for adrenal disease patients. Blood donation acceptance depends on where you live and what organization is accepting blood donations. If you are eligible to donate in your area, remember it is also a personal choice. You should discuss it with your doctor to determine your risks and benefits of blood donation.

## Pregnancy

Though certain forms of adrenal diseases can cause a reduction in fertility, there is outstanding evidence[18] that

---

[15] Donating Blood." The Pituitary Foundation, The Pituitary Foundation - UK National Charity, www.pituitary.org.uk/information/living-with-a-pituitary-condition/donating-blood/.

[16] Target Information Systems Ltd. "JPAC - Transfusion Guidelines." Transfusion Guidelines , JPACJoint United Kingdom (UK) Blood Transfusion and Tissue Transplantation Services Professional Advisory Committee, www.transfusionguidelines.org/dsg/wb/guidelines/ad003-adrenal-failure.

[17] "Blood Donor Eligibility Criteria Alphabetical Listing." Blood Donor Eligibility Criteria | Red Cross Blood Services, The American National Red Cross, www.redcrossblood.org/donate-blood/how-to-donate/eligibility-requirements/eligibility-criteria-alphabetical.html.

[18] Abraham, Mini R. "Adrenal Disease and Pregnancy." Edited by Carl V Smith. Overview, Adrenal Glands in Pregnancy, Renin-Angiotensin-

pregnancy can be successful to full gestation even with the presence of adrenal disease, pending correct glucocorticoid therapy is administered.

The use of dexamethasone should be avoided in pregnant adrenal patients, as it crosses the placenta[19]. Proper stress dosing of cortisol replacement during labor is also essential to sustain the life of an adrenal insufficient mother. Surgical stress dosing considerations must also be considered if a mother requires a cesarean section instead of a vaginal delivery.

Pregnancy can cause some forms of adrenal insufficiency such as:

**Lymphocytic Hypophysitis[20]-** Typically presents in women in late pregnancy or the postpartum period. This condition can cause ACTH deficiency, acute adrenal crisis and isolated growth hormone (GH) deficiency. Presents with symptoms of hyperprolactinemia, headaches, visual disturbances or impairment.

---

Aldosterone System in Pregnancy. American Association of Clinical Endocrinologists, Endocrine Society, November 9, 2019. https://emedicine.medscape.com/article/127772-overview.

[19] Lekarev, Oksana, and Maria I New. "Adrenal Disease in Pregnancy." Best practice & research. Clinical endocrinology & metabolism. U.S. National Library of Medicine, December 2011. https://www.ncbi.nlm.nih.gov/pubmed/22115169.

[20] "Lymphocytic Hypophysitis." Genetic and Rare Diseases Information Center. U.S. Department of Health and Human Services. Accessed April 10, 2020. https://rarediseases.info.nih.gov/diseases/10349/lymphocytic-hypophysitis.

**Sheehan's Syndrome**[21]- Caused by blood loss and hypovolemic shock during or after childbirth resulting in hypopituitarism. Presents with symptoms of inability to produce breastmilk, lack of menstruation, low blood pressure, low blood sugar, increased fatigue and irregular heartbeat.

The most serious concern to an adrenal insufficient woman is low cortisol, which can result in an adrenal crisis. Stress dosing and proper hormone replacement therapy are essential to a successful pregnancy. An adrenal crisis is a sudden, life-threatening event that can lead to shock, coma and death of the mother and likely the fetus if timely medical intervention is not made.

## Alcohol

Arguably, there is no healthcare provider who will suggest consuming alcohol is a good choice for anyone with chronic health issues. Those with endocrine disorders such as adrenal insufficiency must be extra vigilant with alcohol consumption. Alcohol-induced hormonal dysregulations affect the entire body and can negatively impact psychological and behavioral disorders. The Journal of Clinical Endocrinology and Metabolism released a study endorsed by The Endocrine Society which showed evidence[22] that alcohol consumption had a direct impact on cortisol levels. Alcohol consumption can damage liver

---

[21] "Sheehan's Syndrome." Mayo Clinic. Mayo Foundation for Medical Education and Research, November 26, 2019. https://www.mayoclinic.org/diseases-conditions/sheehans-syndrome/symptoms-causes/syc-20351847.
[22] Badrick, Ellena et al. "The relationship between alcohol consumption and cortisol secretion in an aging cohort." The Journal of clinical endocrinology and metabolism vol. 93,3 (2008): 750-7. doi:10.1210/jc.2007-0737

function and reduce the bodies' ability to metabolize cortisol. Impaired inhibitory control of the Hypothalamus-Pituitary-Adrenal axis was also noted in this study. Some adrenal disease patients, especially salt wasting forms, may struggle with electrolyte homeostasis, which can be negatively impacted by alcohol consumption. Alcohol consumption is not recommended in patients with any form of cortisol or aldosterone deficiency.

## Cannabis and CBD

**Cannabinoids**: Derivatives of the cannabis plant. The most commonly used cannabinoid is marijuana.

**THC**: Tetrahydrocannabinol, the most potent bioactive component of cannabinoids. This chemical is what causes psychoactive effects or a "high" with cannabinoid use.

**CBD**: A compound in the class of "phytocannabinoids," which are unique to cannabis plants. Does not contain tetrahydrocannabinol (THC).

On June 25, 2018, the U.S. Food and Drug Administration (FDA) recognized a cannabidiol as a real medicine by approving a medication called Epidiolex. This medication is a pharmaceutical CBD drug used to treat severe pediatric seizures.

Many states in America have legalized[23] the use of Marijuana for medical or recreational use. Decriminalization policies regarding marijuana use are also being adopted nationwide, dependent on each state's laws and jurisdiction. Which begs the question, is CBD's

---

[23] "Map of Marijuana Legality by State." DISA Global Solutions, 2 Apr. 2020, disa.com/map-of-marijuana-legality-by-state.

newfound popularity due to its supposedly amazing results or has enough research been conducted to truly know its short and long-term effects?

There is much debate in the scientific community regarding that very question. The discovery[24] of the Endocannabinoid system (ECS[25]) only added to this discussion. The ECS is the concept that the body itself contains endogenous cannabinoids which are similar to cannabinoids, but they are produced by your body.

**The ECS involves three core components:**

1-Endocannabinoids

2-Receptors

3-Enzymes.

**The body produces two endocannabinoids:**

1-Anandamide (AEA)

2-Arachidonoylglyerol (2-AG)

**The body also contains two main endocannabinoid receptors:**

1-CB1 receptors. Mainly found in the central nervous system.

2-CB2 receptors. Mainly found in the peripheral nervous system and in immune cells.

---

[24] Lee, Martin A. "Https://Www.beyondthc.com/Wp-Content/Uploads/2012/07/ECBSystemLee.pdf." The Discovery of the Endocannabinoid System, The National Institute on Drug Abuse, www.beyondthc.com/wp-content/uploads/2012/07/eCBSystemLee.pdf

[25] Raypole, Crystal. "Endocannabinoid System: A Simple Guide to How It Works." Healthline. Healthline Media, February 13, 2020. https://www.healthline.com/health/endocannabinoid-system#cbd.

**Enzymes are what breaks down the endocannabinoids. There are thought to be two enzymes that perform this function:**

1-Fatty acid amide hydrolase. Breaks down AEA.

2-Monoacylglycerol acid lipase: Breaks down 2-AG.

Cannabis (THC) interacts with your ECS by binding to receptors, just like your natural endocannabinoids. THC binds to both CB1 and CB2 receptors, which can cause a myriad of effects in the body. Cannabis users report side effects such as reduce pain and increased appetite. THC has also been known to cause paranoia and anxiety.

According to Polish Society of Endocrinology[26], "Cannabinoids have been confirmed to deeply impact the endocrine system, including the activity of the pituitary gland, adrenal cortex, thyroid gland, pancreas, and gonads. Interrelations between the endocannabinoid system and the activity of the endocrine system may be a therapeutic target for a number of drugs that have been proved effective in the treatment of infertility, obesity, diabetes, and even prevention of diseases associated with the cardiovascular system."

There is currently little to no research on cannabis and its effects on those with endocrine diseases such as adrenal insufficiency. It is important to discuss any treatment with your healthcare provider and be aware that the CBD market is currently severely unregulated. Do your research before you try any product and be aware that scams do exist. Only

---

[26] Borowska, Magdalena, et al. "The Effects of Cannabinoids on the Endocrine System." Endokrynologia Polska, Polish Society of Endocrinology, 20 Dec. 2018, journals.viamedica.pl/endokrynologia_polska/article/view/58487.

you and your physician can truly decide if CBD products are a good fit for you.

## Hyperbaric Oxygen Therapy

Is hyperbaric oxygen therapy safe with adrenal disease?

Hyperbaric oxygen therapy is an alternative treatment used to promote healing. With this treatment, a patient is placed in a hyperbaric oxygen therapy chamber, in which the air pressure is increased to higher than normal air pressure so that the patient's lungs can absorb more oxygen. The pressurized oxygen expelled within the chamber is believed to help your blood carry more oxygen and therefore promote healing and wellness. Hyperbaric oxygen therapy increases the amount of oxygen the blood can carry. It is believed this increase in blood oxygen temporarily restores normal levels of blood gases and allows tissue function to promote healing and fight infections. Hyperbaric oxygen therapy is considered a generally safe procedure, but this treatment does carry risks for adrenal disease patients.

A study[27] by the Undersea and Hyperbaric Medical Society performed in 2008 revealed the following:
**"The attendant with Addison's disease was found to have a drop from a morning level of 16.5 ug/dl to a critical level of 1.4 ug/dl. Subsequent testing without HBOT showed a lesser, non-critical drop of 29.1ug/dl to 9 ug/dl (normal range for the circadian cycle.)"**

US National Library of Medicine National Institutes of Health also released a study[28] with the following results:

[27] Abstract of the Undersea & Hyperbaric Medical Society 2008 Annual Scientific Meeting June 26-28, 2008 Salt Lake City Marriott Downtown, Salt Lake City, Utah.
http://archive.rubicon-foundation.org/7867

**Cortisol levels decreased significantly (P = 0.001) during the treatments. No significant changes were found in other analyzed hormones.**

It is important to be aware that hyperbaric oxygen therapy has been shown to decrease serum cortisol levels, therefore making this treatment a concern for those with adrenal disease.  If you are a cortisol pump user, you will not be able to have your pump within the hyperbaric chamber to administer your cortisol. Due to the high oxygen concentration, devices are a fire hazard concern. If you are considering hyperbaric oxygen therapy, please consider the above research and thoroughly discuss the risks and benefits of this treatment with your doctor.

# Chapter 7: Upcoming Emergency Cortisol Injection Device

Adrenal disease patients anxiously await the release of the Twistject- Emergency Cortisol Injection Device!

The company, Solution Medical, is developing a one-step injector for delivering adrenal crisis medication in a rescue situation. This incredible innovation will eliminate the need for cumbersome and confusing rescue kits, and replace those kits with a single, one-step device. This upcoming device automatically mixes medication without requiring

---

[28] US National Library of Medicine National Institutes of Health – Effect of hyperbaric conditions on plasma stress hormone levels. Department of Anesthesiology, Turku University Hospital, Finland. https://www.ncbi.nlm.nih.gov/pubmed/10372427

shaking or visual monitoring. Initial data shows the product mixes hydrocortisone sodium succinate powder approximately 20X faster than the current standard of care in only one user step.

Solution's design teams, Neuma and IDE have been focused on the optimization and full integration, assembly, and prototyping of this device and recently finished the first complete prototype integration and demonstration successfully.

With their device prototype, Solution has completed "hands-on" demonstrations with patients and advocacy groups to glean initial feedback from partners, patients, and caregivers. They are also planning to conduct a "human factor" study [2022] with The Children's Hospital of Pennsylvania (CHOP). Having adrenal insufficiency herself, Solution's founder, Julia Anthony, has maintained the focus of the product to be the usability and the human factors aspects of the device.

On their drug formulation effort, they have optimized partners and supply chains and are working with two UK firms – Nova Labs (formulation) and Intertek (analytical) – to deliver the drug to the required specifications. These new formulation partners can offer potential cost/development savings.

Solution Medical was pleased with the promising analytical results of the optimized spray drying formulation and are moving forward with finalizing the formulation for manufacturability.

Solution Medical also completed a pricing and reimbursement strategy and payer stakeholder engagement and were very encouraged by the results, which included interviews with payer pharmacy benefit managers and medical directors. Based on this effort, they expect patients will have full access to the Twistject device across public and private payers, with no restrictions, no step through therapy (i.e. fail other methods first before changing), no prior authorization, and strong reimbursement rates.

Additionally, they are in the process of primary market research with patients and caregivers, to better understand their needs, the number of prescriptions per year, the number of crises per year, and other information relating to current adrenal crisis medication utilization. Solution has had over 400 global survey respondents, which helped them better understand patient and caregiver needs, as well as aid them in payer discussions and negotiations.

Solution Medical continues to expand external relationships and was selected to be part of the NASDAQ Milestone Maker Program, which has already led to several meetings with potential strategic partners for distribution worldwide. This incredible company continues to build momentum and we are excited to support their ongoing efforts to make the Twistject device a reality! For more information, visit their website at: www.solutionmedco.com.

# Chapter 8: Alternative Adrenal Assessment

Author of this book, Winslow E. Dixon spent the last decade working with the organization Adrenal Alternatives Foundation where she worked with stress-related conditions, adrenal diseases and cortisol care. After realizing the limitations western medicine has regarding integrating holistic health into adrenal care, she made the decision to resign from Adrenal Alternatives and open her own naturopathic practice, Hope Healing Happy Clinic. Her clinic's protocols go further than your standard protocols in endocrinology because they look into your cortisol replacement, lifestyle, genetics and stress levels. This chapter discusses her process for helping patients achieve optimal health despite adrenal disease.

## Hope Healing Happy Clinic's Adrenal Protocol

### 1. At Home Adrenal Testing.

The first line, standard testing protocol in western medicine for cortisol care is an 8:00am blood serum cortisol lab. This test evaluates the total serum cortisol levels in a person's body. While it is useful to indicate and diagnose cases of Cushing's and Addison's, it is very limited when trying to evaluate HPA axis dysfunction and managing patients who are already being treated with cortisol replacement. At home cortisol test kits can be a useful tool when trying to establish the correct cortisol replacement dose and timing schedule for adrenal insufficiency patients.

Hope Healing Happy Clinic provides a test kit you can easily perform in the comfort of your own home. The test involves urine, bloodspot and saliva cortisol testing throughout a 24-hour period to get an evaluation of your current adrenal hormone replacement. The test results are the most accurate when a person takes the tests during their normal routine to evaluate how your current cortisol replacement medication dose and schedule are managing your personal, average day-to-day lifestyle.

Proper cortisol replacement is deeply crucial to circadian rhythm modulation and quality of life for adrenal disease patients. Standard oral steroid replacement done incorrectly can render adrenal insufficient patients under or over replaced within the same 24-hour dosing period. We understand that every adrenal patient is different and steroid replacement needs to be tailored to each patient depending on their health status and lifestyle. Though we do not prescribe medications, we work alongside endocrinology professionals to ensure correct cortisol replacement is being administered.

## 2. Lifestyle Assessment.

We perform a detailed lifestyle assessment to understand not only HOW your body reacts but also figuring out WHAT it is reacting to and WHEN. We compare your lab results to the lifestyle assessment, which allows us to have a deeper insight into why you may be struggling with quality of life, energy levels, anxiety, depression, weight management and/or fatigue.

## 3. Define Your Chronotype.

A person's chronotype is defined as their genetic internal master clock which defines circadian rhythm, regulates the sleep-wake cycle and other bodily functions like appetite and temperature. Depending on your specific genes, your body will function in a certain way and produce hormones according to your personal circadian rhythm modulation. Defining your chronotype will help you establish lifestyle changes and set a schedule that works best for your optimal health, energy levels and productivity. We work with patients to discover their personal genomics and create a plan of recovery tailored to their needs.

## 3. Support the Basics.

The goal of adrenal disease management is to replace the right amount of steroid hormones to induce healthy cortisol activities such as a proper sleep/wake cycle and avoid putting your body into a "fight or flight" state.

Adrenal patients are typically great at pushing through pain, exhaustion, and grief. These people are typically strong willed and well accomplished, but they can be terrible at providing their bodies with basic necessities such as: Getting adequate sleep at night, staying hydrated, nourishing their body by eating when they are hungry, resting when they are tired, saying "no" to situations, tasks or favors for others and even breathing properly. These little things truly make a difference in quality of life. We work with patients to reset their circadian rhythm and reduce stress. We also offer a myriad of adjunct, alternative services to support health such as: Biblical meditation, counseling, tuning fork therapy, chromotherapy, frequency medicine and (PEMF) pulsed electromagnetic field therapy.

## 4. Blood Glucose Regulation.

Cortisol, insulin and glucose are cofactors in the body, which basically means one impacts another. Cortisol availability has been implicated in abnormal glucose and fat metabolism. Research[29] has also indicated that diurnal

---

[29] Hackett RA, Kivimäki M, Kumari M, Steptoe A. Diurnal Cortisol Patterns, Future Diabetes, and Impaired Glucose Metabolism in the Whitehall II Cohort Study. J Clin Endocrinol Metab. 2016 Feb;101(2):619-25. doi: 10.1210/jc.2015-2853. Epub 2015 Dec 8. PMID: 26647151; PMCID: PMC4880118.

cortisol secretion is associated with future neuroendocrine dysfunctions is related to the pathophysiology of diabetes, however the mechanisms through which changes in cortisol impairs glucose metabolism are not yet understood. Unfortunately, this means adrenal patients on long term steroid replacement therapy are at increased risk for developing diabetes, which is why healthy glucose levels are a focus in our adrenal management program. Additionally, health "trends" such as intermittent fasting are discouraged in adrenal patients because it can further disrupt the circadian rhythm and can even cause the body to produce adrenaline in response to the stress of not having any "fuel" to function. It is not just about **what** you are eating, but **when** and **how**. We work with our patients to understand how to regulate their blood glucose levels.

## 5. Alternative Medicine.

A noteworthy tool in the fight for adrenal health is the therapeutic use of alternative medicine and holistic modalities such as acupuncture and massage. Many alternative remedies can be greatly beneficial in supporting adrenal health. However, they must be done carefully under the direction of licensed professionals, which is why we have a nurse practitioner and clinical herbalist on our staff who will review all medications and medical conditions to ensure none of them will interact with any natural protocols. It is important to note that no alternative remedies can replace cortisol in the cases of adrenal insufficiency, which requires steroid medications such as: hydrocortisone, prednisone or dexamethasone to sustain life. Again, there is **NO** herbal remedy, natural compound, diet or lifestyle change that will replace cortisol in adrenal insufficiency patients! Alternative medicine and herbalism

https://www.ncbi.nlm.nih.gov/pmc/articles/PMC4880118/

are ways to support the body but will not replace steroid medications. Never discontinue, reduce or change your steroid medications without the advice of an overseeing medical professional.

## 6. Frequency Medicine.

Frequency medicine is the use of electromagnetic resonances, tones, microcurrents and soundwaves to promote the body's natural healing abilities. Your body has a natural frequency that it resonates at. For example, your heart beats and produces a wavelength that can be measured by an EKG. Similarly, all organ systems produce their own frequency. When a cell or organ system becomes damaged, it can disrupt the healthy frequency. When these frequencies become out of balance, symptoms arise. An imbalance in frequency can cause physical, emotional and mental health symptoms.

Ultrasound machines can capture images inside the human body by sending sound waves into a person and collects the ones that bounce back then sends them to a computer to be converted into a physical image. Frequency machines work in a similar way by introducing the correct resonance back into the body. Introducing the body to specific frequencies is like translating the correct language to support an organ's optimal health. Frequency medicine introduces the correct tones to your body to help it self-regulate. Frequencies are simply translating a "language" the body understands.

During the treatment, our practitioner will either use headphones for auditory frequency therapy or attach small probes, similar to a TENS unit machine to deliver physical frequencies into your body. The frequencies used during treatment are extremely mild — one millionth of an ampere. Such a small amount of electrical current is safe because the human body naturally produces its own current within each of your cells.  It is a non-invasive, non-medicinal, highly targeted therapy.  Frequency medicine is used to help the body enter a natural healing state. Precise frequencies can target the direct source and accelerate the body's natural recovery at the cellular level. They are used to reduce pain, inflammation and even emotional healing in a safe, natural way.

Though generally regarded as safe, there are certain groups of people who shouldn't receive Frequency Medicine treatment, including:

- People who have uncontrolled seizures or conditions such as epilepsy.
- People with implanted pumps or other medical devices.
- People with pacemakers.
- People with late-stage cancers.
- Pregnant women.

Frequency medicine is not intended to diagnose, treat or cure any condition and should only be used to support the body's natural ability to heal. Never start any treatment without first consulting your licensed healthcare provider.

**Cortisol Care**

Cortisol care is a fight you must take in stride with patience. In order to heal, you do not need to push harder. You just need to listen to your body and give it what it needs.

If you need adrenal health management, you can schedule a remote or in-person adrenal health assessment at Hope Healing Happy Clinic!  To schedule your consult, book a timeslot on the website, Hopehealinghappy.com or call (941) 841-9903.☐☐☐☐

For more information follow our social media:

TikTok: hopehealinghappy_clinic
Instagram: hopehealinghappyclinic
Facebook.com/hopehealinghappyco
Youtube: youtube.com/@HopeHealingHappy

Adrenal disease certainly presents itself with its own unique challenges, but it is not impossible to live a happy and fulfilling life despite this disease. Proper self-care, medication and stress management are imperative to living the best life possible. My hope is that this book helped provide you with some information that helps you improve your quality of life. I know how difficult it is to battle adrenal disease and all my years in Adrenal Alternatives Foundation showed me that we are all incredible fighters to handle the cortisol battle we do. I wish you hope, healing and happiness. Thanks for reading my book.
Sincerely, Winslow E. Dixon

# Chapter 9: Conclusion

# Sources/References

Acute adrenal crisis (Addisonian Crisis)
Uclahealth.org. (n.d.). Acute Adrenal Crisis - (Addisonian crisis). [online] Available at:
https://www.uclahealth.org/endocrine-center/acute-adrenal-crisis [Accessed 15 Dec. 2019].

Abraham, Mini R. "Adrenal Disease and Pregnancy."
Edited by Carl V Smith, Overview, Adrenal Glands in
Pregnancy, Renin-Angiotensin-Aldosterone System in
Pregnancy, American Association of Clinical
Endocrinologists, Endocrine Society, 9 Nov. 2019,
emedicine.medscape.com/article/127772-overview.

"Blood Donor Eligibility Criteria Alphabetical Listing."
Blood Donor Eligibility Criteria | Red Cross Blood
Services, The American National Red Cross,
www.redcrossblood.org/donate-blood/how-to-
donate/eligibility-requirements/eligibility-criteria-
alphabetical.html.

Borowska, Magdalena, et al. "The Effects of Cannabinoids
on the Endocrine System." Endokrynologia Polska, Polish
Society of Endocrinology, 20 Dec. 2018,
journals.viamedica.pl/endokrynologia_polska/article/view/
58487.

"Donating Blood." The Pituitary Foundation, The Pituitary
Foundation - UK National Charity,
www.pituitary.org.uk/information/living-with-a-pituitary-
condition/donating-blood/.

Hackett RA, Kivimäki M, Kumari M, Steptoe A. Diurnal
Cortisol Patterns, Future Diabetes, and Impaired Glucose
Metabolism in the Whitehall II Cohort Study. J Clin
Endocrinol Metab. 2016 Feb;101(2):619-25. doi:
10.1210/jc.2015-2853. Epub 2015 Dec 8. PMID:
26647151; PMCID: PMC4880118.
https://www.ncbi.nlm.nih.gov/pmc/articles/PMC4880118/

Oldfield EH, et al. Petrosal sinus sampling with and
without corticotropin-releasing hormone for the differential

diagnosis of Cushing's syndrome. N Engl J Med. 1991; 325:897.

Nieman LK, et al. The ovine corticotropin-releasing hormone stimulation test and the dexamethasone suppression test in the differential diagnosis of Cushing's syndrome. Ann Int Med. 1986; 105:862.

Yanovski JA, et al. Corticotropin-releasing hormone stimulation following low-dose dexamethasone administration. JAMA. 1993; 269: 2232.

Chrousos GP, et al. The corticotropin-releasing factor stimulation test: An aid in the evaluation of patients with Cushing's syndrome. N Engl J Med. 1984; 310:622. Endocrine Abstracts 23rd Joint Meeting of the British Endocrine Societies with the European Federation of Endocrine Societies Brighton, UK 22 - 24 Mar 2004 British Endocrine Societies ISSN 1470-3947 (print) | ISSN 1479-6848 (online)© BioScientifica 2020

Berneis K, Staub JJ, Gessler A, et al. Combined stimulation of adrenocorticotropin and compound-S by single dose metyrapone test as an outpatient procedure to assess hypothalamic-pituitary-adrenal function. J Clin Endocrinology Metabolism 2002; 87:5470.

Gibney J, Healy ML, Smith TP, McKenna TJ. A simple and cost-effective approach to assessment of pituitary adrenocorticotropin and growth hormone reserve: combined use of the overnight metyrapone test and insulin-like growth factor-I standard deviation scores. J Clinical Endocrinology Metabolism 2008; 93:3763.

Cortisol Pumping Survey

adrenalalternatives.com. (2020). Cortisol Pumping Survey. [online] Available at: https://docs.google.com/forms/d/1eWYZjIFP9HRJDosvdi mJnOr8p54Rmpx_2A4Xz40f77A/edit#responses [Accessed 8 Jan. 2020].

Replication of cortisol circadian rhythm: new advances in hydrocortisone replacement therapy
Chan, D. and Debono, M. (n.d.). Replication of cortisol circadian rhythm: new advances in hydrocortisone replacement therapy. [online] Therapeutic Advances in Endocrinology and Metabolism. Available at: https://www.ncbi.nlm.nih.gov/pmc/articles/PMC3475279/ [Accessed 13 Dec. 2019].

U.S. Department of Health and Human Services
Information, H., Diseases, E., Disease, A., Causes, S., Causes, S., Center, T. and Health, N. (2020). U.S. Department of Health and Human Services. [online] National Institute of Diabetes and Digestive and Kidney Diseases. Available at: https://www.niddk.nih.gov/health-information/endocrine-diseases/adrenal-insufficiency-addisons-disease/symptoms-causes [Accessed 8 Jan. 2020].

National Sleep Foundation Recommends New Sleep Times | National Sleep Foundation. [online] Available at: https://www.sleepfoundation.org/press-release/national-sleep-foundation-recommends-new-sleep-times [Accessed 5 Jan. 2020].

Prednisone and other corticosteroids: Balance the risks and benefits. [online] Available at:

https://www.mayoclinic.org/steroids/art-20045692
[Accessed 4 Jan. 2020].

Subcutaneous hydrocortisone administration for emergency use in adrenal insufficiency PUBMED – Ncbi.nlm.nih.gov. (2013). Subcutaneous hydrocortisone administration for emergency use in adrenal insufficiency. - PubMed - NCBI. [online] Available at:
https://www.ncbi.nlm.nih.gov/pubmed/23672956
[Accessed 10 Dec. 2019].

Types of adrenal gland disorders (2020). Types of adrenal gland disorders. [online] Available at:
https://www.nichd.nih.gov/health/topics/adrenalgland/conditioninfo/types [Accessed 8 Jan. 2020].

Lee, Martin A.
"Https://Www.beyondthc.com/WpContent/Uploads/2012/07/ECBSystemLee.pdf." The Discovery of the Endocannabinoid System, The National Institute on Drug Abuse, www.beyondthc.com/wp-content/uploads/2012/07/eCBSystemLee.pdf.

Lekarev, Oksana, and Maria I New. "Adrenal Disease in Pregnancy." Best Practice & Research. Clinical Endocrinology & Metabolism, U.S. National Library of Medicine, Dec. 2011,
www.ncbi.nlm.nih.gov/pubmed/22115169.

"Lymphocytic Hypophysitis." Genetic and Rare Diseases Information Center, U.S. Department of Health and Human Services,
rarediseases.info.nih.gov/diseases/10349/lymphocytic-hypophysitis.

"Map of Marijuana Legality by State." DISA Global
Solutions, 2 Apr. 2020, disa.com/map-of-marijuana-
legality-by-state.

"Medical Conditions Affecting Donation." Memorial Sloan
Kettering Cancer Center, www.mskcc.org/about/get-
involved/donating-blood/additional-donor-
requirements/medical-conditions-affecting-donation.

Raypole, Crystal. "Endocannabinoid System: A Simple
Guide to How It Works." Healthline, Healthline Media, 13
Feb. 2020, www.healthline.com/health/endocannabinoid-
system#cbd.

"Sheehan's Syndrome." Mayo Clinic, Mayo Foundation for
Medical Education and Research, 26 Nov. 2019,
www.mayoclinic.org/diseases-conditions/sheehans-
syndrome/symptoms-causes/syc-20351847.

Target Information Systems Ltd. "JPAC - Transfusion
Guidelines." Transfusion Guidelines, JPAC Joint United
Kingdom (UK) Blood Transfusion and Tissue
Transplantation Services Professional Advisory
Committee,www.transfusionguidelines.org/dsg/wb/guidelin
es/ad003-adrenal-failure

# About the Author

Winslow E. Dixon, spent the last decade as the CEO the
organization, Adrenal Alternatives Foundation, where she
worked in cortisol care, advocating for people with various
types of cortisol deficiency and adrenal diseases. Through
the EveryLife Foundation's community congress, she also
volunteered in the Rare Disease Congressional Caucus in

the United States Congress to advocate for legislation that legalized the revolutionary treatment of the cortisol pump in America. (Right to Try Act 2017)

The Right to Try Act allowed eligible patients to request access to certain investigational medical treatments that have not yet been approved by the FDA and allows patients and their doctors work to request access to lifesaving medical options without involving FDA approval.

Winslow has since resigned from nonprofit work and is now a naturopathic practitioner with Hope Healing Happy Clinic. She is also an ordained minister through the Universal Life Church. She sees clients both remotely on zoom and in person at the clinic's Florida location.

Winslow has also published multiple books on the topic of adrenal health including the best sellers, Adrenal Insufficiency 101: A Patient's Guide to Managing Adrenal Insufficiency and Cortisol Pump 101: A Patient's Guide to the Cortisol Pumping Method. She is also in the process of publishing two more books on adrenal disease, Overcoming Addison's which is her personal story and Cortisol Care 101.

Her other published books include:
Arsenal of Arrows Journal Challenge Series
Chronically Stoned: The Guide to Winning the Battle against Kidney Stones and UTI's
Holistic Homemaking: Guide to Identifying Toxic Exposure and Creating Natural Products.
Peace by Piece 365 Inspirational Health Log Journal
The Shivering Sunbeam. Children's book which explains disability in a way young minds can understand.

<u>Townsend</u>: The EverVigilant Series, Fiction Adventure Series. All are available through Amazon, Kindle E-book and Barnes and Noble.

Winslow lives by her mantra, "*When you've been through hell, leave sparks of fire wherever you go.*" ©

Learn more about Winslow on her social media:
youtube.com/@WinslowEDixon
facebook.com/winslowedixon
Website- winslowedixon.com
Instagram- Authorwedixon

# Dedications

This book is dedicated to the incredible spirit of all the adrenal disease warriors who battle this incredibly difficult disease.  Thanks also to the Adrenal Alternatives Foundation, my time with you showed me that the resilience of the human spirit is stronger than any disease ever could be.

Best wishes to the American Adrenal Association who continued our work. Special thanks to Susie Mathis, who is their new CEO as of April 2023. Thanks for picking up the torch I could no longer carry!

www.ingramcontent.com/pod-product-compliance
Lightning Source LLC
Chambersburg PA
CBHW030853270326
41928CB00008B/1356